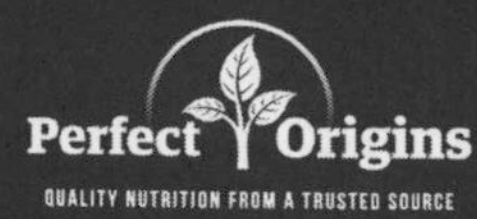

Disclaimer

This book is intended as a reference material, not as a medical manual to replace the advice of your physician or to substitute for any treatment prescribed by your physician.

If you are ill or suspect that you have a medical problem, we strongly encourage you to consult your medical, health, or other competent professional before adopting any of the suggestions in this book or drawing inferences from it. If you are taking prescription medication, you should never change your diet (for better or worse) without consulting your physician, as any dietary change may affect the metabolism of that prescription drug.

This book and the author's opinions are solely for informational and educational purposes.

The author specifically disclaims all responsibility for any liability, loss, or risk, personal or otherwise which is incurred as a consequence, directly or indirectly, of the use and application of any of the contents of this book.

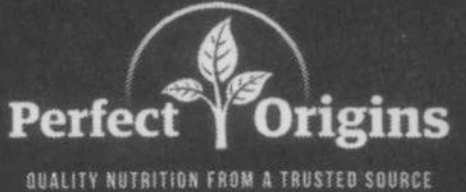

TABLE OF CONTENTS

Read Me First 4

Accountability Contract 6

What's Your Why 8

Goal Setting 10

Measurements 15

7 Day Food and Exercise Log 16

Perfect Origins Perfect Foods 17

My Favorite Recipes 20

My Personal Speedy Grocery List 25

Program Review 31

- #1- Lose 1-2 pounds a week on average 32
- #2- Lose 3 pounds a week on average 33
- #3- Lose 4 pounds a week on average 33

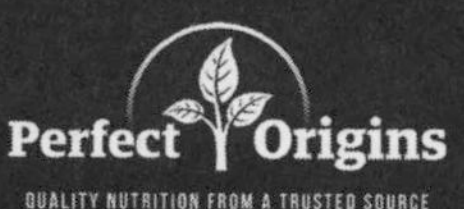

LivLean Formula #1 Protocol and Explanation 35

Daily Lemon Water 50

Master Cleanse (Optional 52

Steps to Perform Master Cleanse 56

Master Cleanse Success Tips 57

Cleansing Side Effects 58

Raw/Alkaline Foods Diet 60

Managing Fruits 69

Structured Eating 70

Cheat Day 77

48-Hour Fast (optional- For those that are hard core ☺) 78

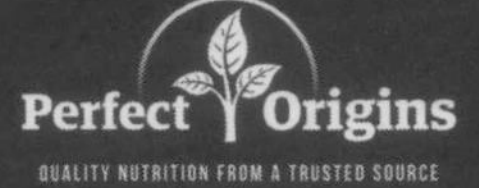

Read Me First

Welcome, Welcome, Welcome! Congratulations on taking that 1st action step to a better, healthier you. I'm not going to bore you with a bunch of words. What I am going to do is give you a bunch of action steps that you can instantly apply to get you started on your fat loss journey. Are you ready?

At Perfect Origins our mission is ... A New You. A Perfect You. A New Beginning. Our mission is to help you on your journey to find the origin of your suffering; be it from weight issues, lack of energy, chronic conditions, or even your vitality.

I only work with people who want to be serious about changing. Through my experience what I've found is that weight loss is only temporary. Lifestyle change is permanent. That's what you want, right? You don't want to keep yo-yo-ing up and down with your weight like you have been do you? Good. I don't want that for you either. It's easier to make a couple simple changes and keep the weight off for good.

Now, you've decided to take action and buy this. What's the next step? It's making the commitment to change. Another a-ha moment for me was when I discovered the phrase "if you think it, you ink it". It means that if you write it down and you will always have better results.

I personally feel that God honors those who are vocal and clear about their goals in life. I find there is something very powerful about writing things down. If you don't believe me, just try it out! I would love to hear your success story!

Below, I've created a contract. The funny thing about this is that as silly as it may seem to sign and date it, there becomes an accountability factor attached to it. Whenever I sign something I instantly feel more accountable than if I just say I'm going to do it.

Go ahead and show this to your friends and family to have them hold you accountable also. Make the promise that you'll stick through this even when times are rough.

Tape this to your bathroom mirror and read it out loud to yourself one time per week and every single time you feel like giving you.

I believe in you. Now it's your turn to believe in yourself!

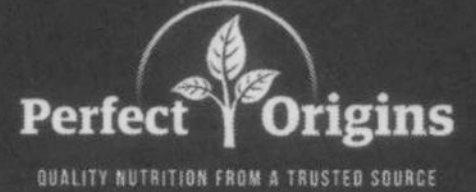

Accountability Contract

I, ________________________________, make this promise to myself and my loved ones that I will complete the Perfect Origins program even though at times it may seem difficult. This includes:

1. Diet: If I cannot complete the cleanse, I will move onto the raw diet, if I cannot complete the raw diet, I will move onto the structured eating portion of the program.

2. I will give myself at least 75 days on this program because I realize that I deserve to live a better, healthier, lifestyle and I recognize that it takes time to develop a healthy habit.

3. I will NOT beat myself up if I cheat or have a moment of weakness. I will just continue the program as is and keep moving forward.

4. I agree that I will never see myself as a failure because there is no such thing as failure, just feedback. I choose to pay attention to my weak points and find ways to overcome them.

5. I will not give up again like I have in so many other programs without discussing this with at least one other person and contacting customer support if I get stuck.

6. I will make sure that I follow through with what I say that I'm going to do because I am a powerful person who takes action.

7. I will remember why I'm doing this program, especially when I'm tempted to stop doing it because it seems "too hard". I will also take control of my thoughts so that my emotions won't dictate my actions.

Signed______________________Date__________

What's Your Why?

In my professional opinion, the major reason why people do not succeed on their diets is because their WHY isn't big enough. Your WHY is the real reason you want to lose weight. This is often underneath the surface stuff such as "I want to fit into my skinny jeans again" or "I want to look good in my bikini". These are much, much deeper. They deal with the more emotional aspects of your life, the suffering, the insecurities, and the embarrassment that you feel. If you can access these deep reasons then you will have found your ultimate motivation.

Let me take a moment and share my personal experience with this. When I connected with my reason why, it felt so much bigger than me. I literally felt like I had to accomplish this no matter what. My WHY for losing my weight was to set an example for my 7 year old son. I wanted him to know that his health was important. I realized that the only way to do this was to BE the example. He watched me make healthy food choices, he exercised with me, he watched me exert will power when I walked by my favorite ice cream shop.

My proudest moment came when he could make his own healthy food choices and when he would ask me to exercise with him. That's powerful.

So let's find out your why. Set the clock for 10 minutes and start writing down the reasons why you want to lose weight. After you clear out the surface reasons, which are a great start, you'll be able to dig deeper to find your WHY.

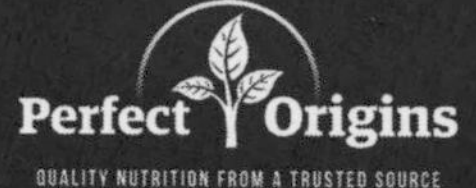

Once you find those reasons that motivate you, then circle them!

The Reason WHY I want to lose weight is:____________

Once you have found your WHY, come back to it and review it every week to keep you focused and motivated!

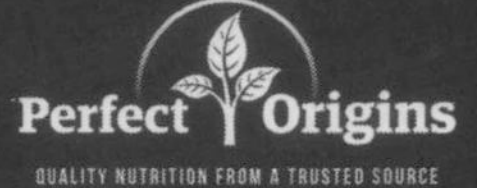

Goal Setting

If you don't know where you are going, you will never get there. The most successful people in life set goals. Now, Perfect Origins is all about creating an easy, fun lifestyle where you can look great, feel great and be able to keep the weight off for good. That's what you want right? In order to get to that point, it's necessary to set goals along the way to move you forward on your journey.

Use this worksheet to help you set a SMART goal.

1. Why do YOU want to adopt a healthier lifestyle?

I want to improve my health because:

____

____

____

____

____

____

____

____

2. Where are you going to start?

I will begin by making a change in the area of:

3. What do you want to accomplish? What is your goal? Is it SMART?

S = Specific

M = Measurable

A = Attainable

R = Relevant

T = Timely

I would like to accomplish the following:

4. How are you going to reach this goal?

During the next week, then month, I will do the following:

5. When are you going to start?

Create a schedule for this week:

Activity Day of the Week Time of Day

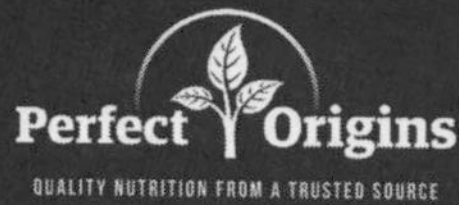

6. Who can help you?

I am going to ask for help from the following people:

7. How will you maintain this change over time? What barriers will interfere with your efforts to maintain the change? What kinds of strengths, supports, and rewards will help you combat those barriers?

Barriers:

Solutions:

My reward for accomplishing my goal is:

If I do not achieve my goal, I will:

When you pick your reward for accomplishing your goal, you should pick something above and beyond what you'd normally do for yourself. Make it big. Go on a trip that you've been wanting to go on. Buy yourself a new wardrobe, give yourself a spa day. Spend more on yourself than normal. You deserve it!

If you do not reach your goal, pick something that you would not enjoy doing, such as cleaning out the garage for your spouse, or taking out the trash for a month. A more constructive idea would be to volunteer at the local soup kitchen for a month. The point is to pick something that will not be convenient for you.

Measurements

It is vital that you measure your success. The best way to do this is by tracking your weight and body measurements.

What you do NOT want to do is just rely on the scale and your weight.

DON'T be a slave to the scale!! It's just one factor to look at. NOT the only one which is a mistake that most people make.

7 Day Food and Exercise Log

The Food and Exercise Log is a critical step in the Perfect Origins program. I find that it is very important to track your eating and exercise habits for a week. Fill this out as complete as you can and look for patterns.

How much are you sleeping? You should be around 7-8 hours a night. How much are you exercising? 3-4 times a week is ideal. How many bowel movements? At least 1 per day. 2-3 is what we strive for. This is a gauge for your fiber intake.

By looking at your past, you can find tiny areas that can be improved without much effort. For example, if you found out that you are drinking 3 sodas a day, drop it down to one and drink green tea in place of the other 2 sodas. This alone would cause you to lose belly fat.

The more you eliminate **wheat, dairy, and sugar** from your diet, the faster you will lose weight. Pay particular attention to those types of foods and focus on eliminating as much as possible. You can do it!

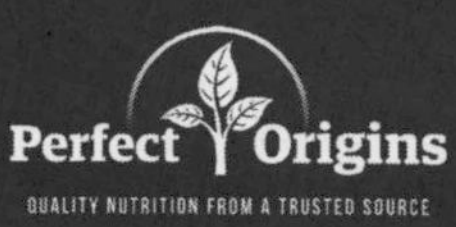

Perfect Origins Perfect Foods

I learned something very interesting during my research and experimenting with myself. I learned that we eat the same basic foods over and over again and that typically, we have about 15 different meals that we eat. Take a moment and think about it... I bet you are just like me and you eat the same things over and over again.

There is nothing wrong with this, especially if you eat healthy foods.

By pre-planning these foods, we are setting ourselves up for success. You can always refer back to this and pick out your "go to" foods. One of the biggest complaints I get in my office is "I don't know what to eat"

We can overcome this by writing it down!

My Favorite Meats/Eggs:

____

____

____

____

____

____

____

____

My Favorite Fats/Oils:

My Favorite Fruits:

My Favorite Vegetables:

My Favorite Nuts/Seeds:

My Favorite Recipes

Thanks to the invention of the internet, you now have access to 100's of different recipes online. The one problem that I can see with this is that it may become overwhelming. So, let's go ahead and write down a few of your favorites.

There are a couple of ways to do this. You can copy and paste them into your own document or you can write down the title and page numbers below.

Raw Food Recipes:

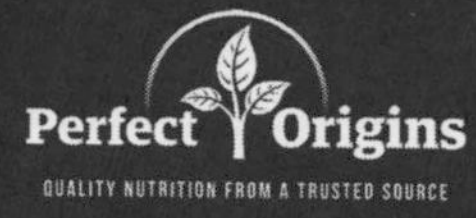

Breakfast Recipes:

Lunch Recipes:

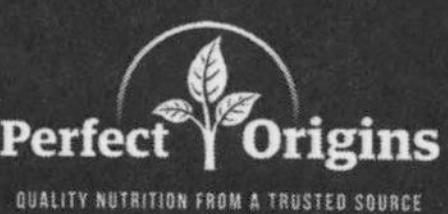

Dinner Recipes:

Snack Recipes:

Smoothie Recipes:

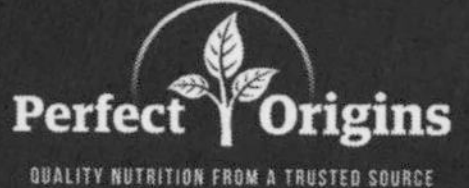

My Personal Speedy Grocery List

Here is a quick list of items that I keep on hand for quick and easy meals. I highly recommend foods that are fresh but I also understand that time is not our friend sometimes ;-) My solution? I find quality frozen produce and meats to keep on hand when I'm in a hurry.

Protein:

Frozen chicken breasts

Frozen turkey burgers (unseasoned)

Frozen wild caught salmon

Frozen cod

Lean ground beef that is antibiotic and hormone free

Cage free eggs

Carbs:

Sweet potatoes/yams

Basmati rice/white rice

Oats

Quinoa

Canned black beans (unseasoned)

Veggies:

Spring mix greens

Spinach

Frozen stir fry veggie mix

Frozen broccoli

Frozen green beans

Fruits:

Green apples

Oranges

Grapes

Lemons

Grapefruits

Frozen berry mix

Fats:

Coconut oil

Extra virgin olive oil

Grass fed butter

Nuts:

Raw almonds

Raw walnuts

Seeds:

Hemp seeds

Pumpkin seeds

Chia Seeds

Beverages:

Filtered water or spring water

Vitamin Water Zero (sweetened with Eryithritol)

Herbal teas

Organic fair trade coffee

Almond milk (unsweetened)

Coconut milk (unsweetened)

Hemp milk (fantastic mixed with coffee)

Mix of Almond/coconut milk unsweetened (my personal favorite)

Condiments:

No salt seasonings such as Mrs. Dash

Sea salt

Dried herbs

Frank's Hot Sauce

Ketchup with no HFCS (high fructose corn syrup)

Cinnamon

Honey (limited amount)

Maple syrup (limited amount)

Supplements:

LivLean Formula #1

Protein Powder

Perfect Biotics

Digestive Enzymes

Greens Powder

BioTRUST Protein Cookies

Perfect Omega TG

Perfect Flush

I am a huge supporter of Biotrust products. I even sit on their scientific advisory board. Personally, I use multiple products of theirs every single day on top of taking the LivLean Supplement, Perfect Biotics, and Perfect Omega TG. Remember that these supplements are optional, but will speed your success. There is no pressure to buy. You can check them out here if you are interested: http://perfectorigins.biotrust.com

Fantastic products, superior quality, and great price!

This is just a reminder if you came to my house right now, the list above is what you'd find. These are my "go to" foods or what I keep around regularly. Yours will be different ☺

The next part of this guide is the actual program overview. When you pick apart the program, it breaks down like this:

Phase 1: Liver/Colon Cleanse

Phase 2: Raw Food Diet

Phase 3: Structured Eating

All three of these are fantastic for your liver and will turn it into the fat burning organ that it should be. You can do all 3 phases which I would highly recommend at least once, or mix and match. The beauty of this program is that it is customizable to you. Go at your own pace if you need to. After all, how do we eat an elephant? One bite at a time!

Just know that my team and I are here to love and support you. We know that you can do it.

Finally, remember that this is designed to be a lifestyle diet. This is exactly what I still do and have been for years. It works at helping you to lose fat, and it helps you to keep it off. And YES I still get to have my ice cream and pizza! After being on this program for a while, my body is conditioned to burn off those goodies fast. Now, I don't eat these all the time, but if I have a craving, I go for it. (Usually about once a week ☺)

THIS is what lifestyle is all about. I don't feel restricted, I don't feel like I can't have something. I make healthy choices and I also get to have my goodies also! You can have this too. I encourage you to stick with me for 90 days even if it is just the structured eating portion. I am confident that you'll have more energy, more focus, more time back and more weight lost than ever before!

Are you ready? Did you get your forms filled out above? Please make sure you give your 110% effort and really try. That includes filling out those papers ;-)

Let's move onto the program breakdown.

Program Overview

In this *Quick Start Guide*, I present three simple plans:

Steady Weight Loss Plan: Lose Approximately 1 to 2 pounds a week on average
Quick Weight Loss Plan: Lose Approximately 3 pounds a week on average
Turbo Weight Loss Plan: Lose Approximately 4 pounds a week on average

Each plan is represented by a color-coded calendar, with each calendar providing a detailed schedule for that plan. After presenting the plan calendars, I explain each part of the diet and give you a brief overview of why it works and why it is beneficial to you.

Note: When reading the average weight loss per week, realize that each week you will not lose that amount. This would be an average over 12 week plan.

Pick Your Weight Loss Plan

Take a moment and consider your weight loss goals. How many pounds do you want to lose? How quickly do you want / need to lose the weight? For example, if you want to lose 20 pounds in three weeks, you should focus on the *Turbo Weight Loss Plan*. However if you are OK with losing 20 pounds over the next three to six months, and you want to enjoy more of the foods you love, then the *Steady Weight Loss Plan* will work just fine.

So let's take a look at the plans…

Steady Weight Loss Calendar

Steady Weight Loss Calendar

	MON	TUES	WED	THURS	FRI	SAT	SUN
WEEK 1	12 PM - 9 PM Structured Eating	12 PM - 9 PM Structured Eating	12 PM - 9 PM Structured Eating	12 PM - 9 PM Structured Eating	12 PM - 9 PM Structured Eating	Cheat Day Stop Eating at 9 PM	12 PM - 9 PM Structured Eating
WEEK 2	12 PM - 9 PM Structured Eating	12 PM - 9 PM Structured Eating	12 PM - 9 PM Structured Eating	12 PM - 9 PM Structured Eating	12 PM - 9 PM Structured Eating	Cheat Day Stop Eating at 9 PM	12 PM - 9 PM Structured Eating
WEEK 3	12 PM - 9 PM Structured Eating	12 PM - 9 PM Structured Eating	12 PM - 9 PM Structured Eating	12 PM - 9 PM Structured Eating	12 PM - 9 PM Structured Eating	Cheat Day Stop Eating at 9 PM	12 PM - 9 PM Structured Eating
WEEK 4	12 PM - 9 PM Structured Eating	12 PM - 9 PM Structured Eating	12 PM - 9 PM Structured Eating	12 PM - 9 PM Structured Eating	12 PM - 9 PM Structured Eating	Cheat Day Stop Eating at 9 PM	12 PM - 9 PM Structured Eating

Quick Weight Loss Calendar

Quick Weight Loss Calendar

	MON	TUES	WED	THURS	FRI	SAT	SUN
WEEK 1	AM - Lemon Water Raw/Alkaline Foods Diet - no time restriction	AM - Lemon Water Raw/Alkaline Foods Diet - no time restriction	AM - Lemon Water Raw/Alkaline Foods Diet - no time restriction	AM - Lemon Water Raw/Alkaline Foods Diet - no time restriction	AM - Lemon Water Raw/Alkaline Foods Diet - no time restriction	AM - Lemon Water Raw/Alkaline Foods Diet - no time restriction	AM - Lemon Water Raw/Alkaline Foods Diet - no time restriction
WEEK 2	AM - Lemon Water 12 PM - 9 PM Structured Eating	AM - Lemon Water 12 PM - 9 PM Structured Eating	AM - Lemon Water 12 PM - 9 PM Structured Eating	AM - Lemon Water 12 PM - 9 PM Structured Eating	AM - Lemon Water 12 PM - 9 PM Structured Eating	Cheat Day Stop Eating at 9 PM	Fast Until 6 PM
WEEK 3	AM - Lemon Water 12 PM - 9 PM Structured Eating	AM - Lemon Water 12 PM - 9 PM Structured Eating	AM - Lemon Water 12 PM - 9 PM Structured Eating	AM - Lemon Water 12 PM - 9 PM Structured Eating	AM - Lemon Water 12 PM - 9 PM Structured Eating	Cheat Day Stop Eating at 9 PM	Fast Until 6 PM
WEEK 4	AM - Lemon Water 12 PM - 9 PM Structured Eating	AM - Lemon Water 12 PM - 9 PM Structured Eating	AM - Lemon Water 12 PM - 9 PM Structured Eating	AM - Lemon Water 12 PM - 9 PM Structured Eating	AM - Lemon Water 12 PM - 9 PM Structured Eating	Cheat Day Stop Eating at 9 PM	Fast Until 6 PM

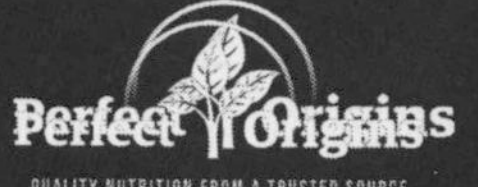

Turbo Weight Loss Calendar

Turbo Weight Loss Calendar

	MON	TUES	WED	THURS	FRI	SAT	SUN
WEEK 1	AM - Lemon Water Raw/Alkaline Foods Diet - no time restriction	AM - Lemon Water Raw/Alkaline Foods Diet - no time restriction	AM - Lemon Water Raw/Alkaline Foods Diet - no time restriction	AM - Lemon Water Raw/Alkaline Foods Diet - no time restriction	AM - Lemon Water Raw/Alkaline Foods Diet - no time restriction	AM - Lemon Water Raw/Alkaline Foods Diet - no time restriction	AM - Lemon Water Raw/Alkaline Foods Diet - no time restriction
WEEK 2	AM - Lemon Water Raw/Alkaline Foods Diet - no time restriction	AM - Lemon Water Raw/Alkaline Foods Diet - no time restriction	AM - Lemon Water Raw/Alkaline Foods Diet - no time restriction	AM - Lemon Water Raw/Alkaline Foods Diet - no time restriction	AM - Lemon Water Raw/Alkaline Foods Diet - no time restriction	AM - Lemon Water Raw/Alkaline Foods Diet - no time restriction	AM - Lemon Water Raw/Alkaline Foods Diet - no time restriction *PM - HERBAL LAXATIVE TEA*
WEEK 3	MASTER CLEANSE *AM - Saltwater Flush 8 glasses of Cleanse Lemonade PM - Herbal Laxative Tea*	MASTER CLEANSE *AM - Saltwater Flush 8 glasses of Cleanse Lemonade PM - Herbal Laxative Tea*	MASTER CLEANSE *AM - Saltwater Flush 8 glasses of Cleanse Lemonade*	AM - Lemon Water Raw/Alkaline Foods Diet - no time restriction	AM - Lemon Water Raw/Alkaline Foods Diet - no time restriction	AM - Lemon Water Raw/Alkaline Foods Diet - no time restriction	MASTER CLEANSE *AM - Saltwater Flush 8 glasses of Cleanse Lemonade PM - Herbal Laxative Tea*
WEEK 4	MASTER CLEANSE *AM - Saltwater Flush 8 glasses of Cleanse Lemonade PM - Herbal Laxative Tea*	MASTER CLEANSE *AM - Saltwater Flush 8 glasses of Cleanse Lemonade*	AM - Lemon Water Raw/Alkaline Foods Diet - no time restriction	AM - Lemon Water Raw/Alkaline Foods Diet - no time restriction	AM - Lemon Water Raw/Alkaline Foods Diet - no time restriction	AM - Lemon Water Raw/Alkaline Foods Diet - no time restriction	AM - Lemon Water Raw/Alkaline Foods Diet - no time restriction
WEEK 5	AM - Lemon Water 12 PM - 9 PM Structured Eating	AM - Lemon Water 12 PM - 9 PM Structured Eating	AM - Lemon Water 12 PM - 9 PM Structured Eating	AM - Lemon Water 12 PM - 9 PM Structured Eating	AM - Lemon Water 12 PM - 9 PM Structured Eating	Cheat Day Stop Eating at 9 PM	Fast Until 6 PM
WEEK 6	AM - Lemon Water 12 PM - 9 PM Structured Eating	AM - Lemon Water 12 PM - 9 PM Structured Eating	AM - Lemon Water 12 PM - 9 PM Structured Eating	AM - Lemon Water 12 PM - 9 PM Structured Eating	AM - Lemon Water 12 PM - 9 PM Structured Eating	Cheat Day Stop Eating at 9 PM	Fast Until 6 PM
WEEK 7	AM - Lemon Water 12 PM - 9 PM Structured Eating	AM - Lemon Water 12 PM - 9 PM Structured Eating	AM - Lemon Water 12 PM - 9 PM Structured Eating	AM - Lemon Water 12 PM - 9 PM Structured Eating	AM - Lemon Water 12 PM - 9 PM Structured Eating	Cheat Day Stop Eating at 9 PM	Fast Until 6 PM
WEEK 8	AM - Lemon Water 12 PM - 9 PM Structured Eating	AM - Lemon Water 12 PM - 9 PM Structured Eating	AM - Lemon Water 12 PM - 9 PM Structured Eating	AM - Lemon Water 12 PM - 9 PM Structured Eating	AM - Lemon Water 12 PM - 9 PM Structured Eating	Cheat Day Stop Eating at 9 PM	Fast Until 6 PM

NOTE: On Fasting days after cheat days, you can eat after 6pm until 9pm.

That depends on you! You can keep doing the structured eating protocol for as long as you like. I personally do this 90% of the time, and the other 10% do what I want which includes eating pancakes and bacon and eggs for breakfast.

Or continue on any other diet plan you would like.

Remember: YOU WILL GAIN WEIGHT BACK if you go right back to your old habits of eating. LivLean Formula #1 is NOT a magical weight loss pill. It is a powerful health supplement that may support your metabolism by helping your liver be more efficient. It also has many other health benefits as listed on the next pages.

Just to be clear: There are no magical weight loss pills. There are health supplements that can help a beat up body to work more efficiently. Paired with the right diet and exercise plan, you can turn your body and health around 180 degrees.

LivLean Formula #1 Protocol and Explanation

For each plan, be sure to take 2 capsules everyday either during the first meal of the day or if you prefer you can take one at your first meal and one with your second.

This product **should be taken with all phases** of the program which includes:

During the master cleanse

During the raw food alkaline diet

During the structured eating diet

During fasting

Let's look more specifically at the particular blend in this product and why it is so powerful for cleansing your liver, and burning fat while enhancing your overall health.

Powerful Ingredient #1: Silybum Marianum

The first ingredient in our blend is Silybum Marianum Seed Extract, better known as milk thistle. This powerful herb hails from the Mediterranean countries and has an active ingredient called Silymarin, which is what provides the key benefits.

Used medicinally for over 2,000 years, Milk thistle has been reported to protect the liver, aids in regeneration of liver cells, and greatly improves liver function. It is typically used to treat liver cirrhosis, chronic hepatitis, toxin-induced liver damage, fatty liver and disorders of the gall bladder. When the liver isn't sluggish and functions properly, it is turned into the fat burning organ that it was designed to be.

But...

A recent study in the Journal of Medicinal Food backs up a new use for milk thistle in type 2 diabetes. In this trial, researchers studied the effect of the herb in patients with long-standing diabetes that wasn't controlled well by diet or the drug glibenclamide.[3] This study also lasted four months and the participants in the silymarin group took 200 mg/day. And like the other study, the average fasting blood glucose fell by 20 percent in the herbal group. Glycated hemoglobin fell by 16 percent. Changes in the placebo group were negligible. The silymarin patients also, quite surprisingly, lost weight. Body mass index (BMI) values fell significantly-by as much as 9 percent: The milk thistle appeared to cause an average weight loss of around 18 lbs.

But there's even more good news from this particular trial. The researchers found that the spike in blood glucose that occurs within four hours of a meal was **lowered by a massive 37 percent** in patients taking the silymarin, compared to a **significant 19 percent rise** in the placebo group.

Let's make this easier to understand... Milk Thistle helps to support not only liver function and detoxification. It also can lower blood glucose which will burn more fat. Now, Combined with sulphur containing amino acids such as N-Acetyl Cysteine which is also in LivLean Formula 1, your liver will burn fat even more efficiently and thus help with your weight control.

[3] Hussain SA. "Silymarin as an adjunct to glibenclamide therapy improves long-term and postprandial glycemic control and body mass index in type 2 diabetes." *J Med Food* 2007; 10(3): 543-547

Selenium

Selenium is a trace mineral that is found in the soil and offers strong protection to the liver as well. It's a mineral involved in many different body processes including the thyroid, liver, spleen, and pancreas, so having this ingredient in the product will help out in a variety of different ways.

Selenium helps the liver to deal with fats in the body and then export them via the bile for elimination. Selenium is a mineral vital for the conversion of the thyroid hormone T4 to its active form T3. It will therefore help those with weight problems due to an under-active thyroid gland or thyroid resistance.

Common symptoms of an under active thyroid gland are as fatigue, muscle weakness, easy weight gain, depression and scalp hair loss.

The form of selenium in LivLean Formula #1 is SelenoExcell. This patented formula is the ONLY certified 100% organically bound High Selenium Yeast standardized with the National Cancer Institute, and it has been selected as the sole intervention agent in a series of cancer prevention and health-related trials. SelenoExcell has been also shown in a Gold-Standard clinical trial published in Journal of American Medical Association (JAMA) to reduce lung, colon, and prostate cancer incidence by 50 - 63 %. SelenoExcell is unique in that it is a supplement backed by pharmaceutical grade research.

http://newhope360.com/regulatory/selenoexcell-receives-coveted-gras-designation

Turmeric

Turmeric is quickly becoming recognized as a fountain of youth "superspice" with near-miraculous potential in modern medicine.

A cohort of scientific studies published in recent years have shown that taking turmeric on a regular basis can actually lengthen lifespan and improve overall quality of life.

This anti-oxidant is known for its numerous anti-cancer properties and an impressive ability to **positively influence over 586 diseases** according to peer-reviewed research from leading universities, turmeric may also be one of the most powerful substances when it comes to **healthy fat loss**. Over 1,543 scientific journal entries are now centered on turmeric's beneficial properties.

Researchers from the Department of Internal Medicine in the University of Texas noted that when rats were fed high doses of this antioxidant, they showed greater activation of enzymes involved with detoxification of the liver tissues.

A recent animal study showed the hypolipidemic effects of curcumin, demonstrating its ability to significantly lower triglycerides and free fatty acids (3). This is a promising result, suggesting curcumin's potential for treating obesity and associated diseases. In another animal study, dietary therapy resulted in significant weight loss and a potential for increasing basal metabolic rate.

More than 13 other peer-reviewed studies have also reached similar conclusions, finding that turmeric intake is directly associated with increased healthy fat loss and decreased insulin issues. What's more, the spice does not come with the harsh side effects that come along with the use-of-historically-dangerous-diet-drugs.

Picorohiza Kurroa 100:1 Root Extract

Picorohiza Kurroa 100:1 Root Extract is an important herb in the traditional Chinese and Ayurvedic systems of medicine, used to treat liver and acts as a very powerful anti-inflammatory agent in the body. In addition to that, it also serves as an antioxidant and can assist with bringing up liver enzymes to appropriate levels.

This root can also help to prevent liver toxicity from building, boosting overall detoxification efforts.

The special patented blend in LivLean Formula #1 called Picroliv according to a 2012 study in The Journal of Pharmacology and Pharmacotherapeutics, supports the use of these active phytochemicals against toxic liver injury, which may act by preventing lipid peroxidation, augmenting the antioxidant defense system or by regenerating the hepatocytes.

Alpha Lipoic Acid

Alpha Lipoic Acid is a fatty acid that is found in all the cells in the body and is required in order for the body to properly produce energy for everyday body functions. In addition to that, it also serves as an antioxidant in the body and can help to recycle the antioxidants of vitamin C and glutathione as well.

An exciting new double-blind trial involving 360 overweight individuals demonstrated that **the group taking Alpha Lipoic Acid lost significantly more weight** (2.1%) than the group taking a placebo, within a 20-week period. [1] Another study involving 1,127 subjects found Lipoic Acid to be an ideal antioxidant supplement for the therapy of overweight conditions. The subjects in this study, both men and women, experienced a significant weight loss of 8%. [2]

2. Alpha-lipoic acid supplementation: a tool for obesity therapy, Carbonelli MG, et al, *Curr Pharm* Des, 16(7):840-6, 2010.

The combination of ALA, silymarin (from milk thistle), and selenium has been shown to replenish glutathione stores, promotes liver cell regeneration, and puts the brakes on viral replication.

N-Acetyl-Cysteine

Next we have N-Acetyl-Cysteine, which is derived from the amino acid L-cysteine. This amino acid is the primary building block for glutathione.

One of glutathione's best-known roles is to defend the cell it inhabits against damage from wastes and toxins. Since the hepatic cells of those with chronic liver disease are consistently stressed as they deflect poisons, the cells' quantity of glutathione becomes even more important.

Glutathione levels decline naturally as people age, fight a chronic disease or are exposed to excessive amounts of toxins. Insufficient glutathione levels reduce the liver's ability to break down drugs, chemicals and other toxins, enhancing the probability of liver damage. Several studies document the role glutathione depletion plays in advancing liver disease.

Even used as an emergency medicine tactic, one of glutathione's building blocks has been extensively revered for protecting the liver from damaging toxins. and can be used for a wide number of different disease and health conditions such as stroke, kidney disease, heart attack, lung cancer, chronic fatigue, and most importantly, liver damage.

"No other antioxidant is as important to overall health as glutathione. It is the regulator and regenerator of immune cells and the most valuable detoxifying agent in the human body. Low levels are associated with hepatic dysfunction, immune dysfunction, cardiac disease, premature aging, and death." *The Immune System Cure*, Lorna R. Vanderhaeghe & Patrick J.D. Bouic, Ph.D.

Choline

Choline is a micronutrient that has been shown to have a lipotropic effect, meaning it promotes the body's use of fat and may help the liver dispose of "trapped" fats.

That helps to prevent the trapping of fats in the liver, as reported by Oregon State University, which could then go on to cause a number of problems associated with the kidney such as jaundice and atherosclerosis as well as the liver including cirrhosis, hepatitis, and toxic liver damage.

Choline works synergistically with inositol, to shuttle fat produced in the liver or fat eaten in our diets, to be burned for energy by our cells. Thus, if we lack these nutrients, it impairs our ability to take fat out of our liver and send it into the blood stream to be excreted or used to make energy.

Artichoke Leaf Extract

While you can simply eat artichokes in your diet regularly, the benefits this food provides are far more potent in extract form with a proprietary blend.

The extracts contain active compounds, caffeoylquinic acids or cynarin, which can be found in the highest concentrations in artichoke leaves and heart. These active substances work in:

- Preventing the buildup of fat and toxins in the body mainly concentrated in the liver
- Reducing the formation of gallstones during the process of weight loss
- Promoting an increase in the beneficial bacteria that can be found in the intestines
- Increasing bile secretion, thus acting like a laxative

A number of animal studies suggest that artichoke protects the liver from damage by chemical toxins.

Boldo Leaf Extract

Boldo was employed in Chilean and Peruvian folk medicine and recognized as an herbal remedy in a number of pharmacopoeias, mainly for the treatment of liver ailments

Boldo is useful in maintaining overall liver health. In the past, Boldo has eased hepatitis, gallstones and jaundice. Boldo also treats liver disease and acts as a cholagogue, assisting in the excretion of bile from the gallbladder.

Burdock Root Extract

This root extract contains chemicals that help it to fight against activity caused by bacteria as well as inflammation and has been used traditional for a wide variety of natural treatments including treating colds, gastrointestinal complaints, joint pain, bladder infections, as well as liver disease.

In *Healing with Whole Foods* Paul Pitchford writes, "Burdock is a virtual cure-all for conditions of *excess*, and significantly purifies the blood while reducing fat and regulating blood sugar.

In one study published by the Journal of Biomedical Science, taking Burdock three times per day showed vast improvements in alleviating hepato-toxicity due to its antioxidant properties. In addition to this, it was also demonstrated to relieve oxidative stress of the liver cells.

The African Journal of Biotechnology concluded that BRE is beneficial in controlling the blood glucose level, improves the lipid metabolism and prevents diabetic complications from lipid peroxidation in experimental diabetic rats.

Dandelion Root Extract

Dandelion Root Extract is the next component of our powerful liver formula and is a very good source of both beta-carotene as well as potassium. This herb will also provide antioxidant benefits in the body and can help to lower the levels of inflammation present while also killing off invading bacteria.

Because of its iron content, Dandelion root is widely used as a remedy for liver ailments, and its diuretic effect can help rid the liver of toxins. Thus, dandelion roots are used for liver and gall bladder detoxification.

Dandelion roots have had a reputation as being effective in promoting weight loss. Laboratory tests on mice and rats had indicated that there was a loss of up to 30% of body weight in 30 days when the animals were fed dandelion extract with their food.

Yellow Dock Root

Finally, wrapping up the list of ingredients in this mix is yellow dock,

Traditionally, yellow dock root has been thought to be a blood purifier and general detoxifier, especially for the liver.

Yellow dock root stimulates bile production, which helps digestion, particularly of fats. Yellow dock root can stimulate a bowel movement to help remove lingering waste from your intestinal tract; it also increases the frequency of urination to assist in toxin elimination. Maintaining an efficient rate of waste elimination can help prevent toxins from accumulating in the liver, and digestive enzymes as well.

Together, this powerful and unique combination of ingredients is going to provide optimal liver health and care.

Vitamin C

Vitamin C functions as an antioxidant and prevents or lessens toxic damage to liver cells. High amounts of vitamin C also have been known to "clean out" the liver, flushing away fats and fatty buildup, protecting the liver against cirrhosis.

Vitamin B 6

Vitamin B6 helps with weight loss through a stimulating effect on the thyroid and by reducing water retention. When calorie intake is low, Vitamin B6 helps convert stored carbohydrates to glucose to maintain normal blood sugar levels.

Folic Acid

Functions to maintain stable levels of insulin together with vitamin B12 and vitamin C. Keeping your blood insulin levels constant is important for efficient fat burning.

Vitamin B 12

Cobalamin or Vitamin B12 helps to increase metabolism, gives a boost of energy and helps to fight stress and depression. The liver stores vitamin B-12. Some evidence suggests a lack of vitamin B-12 causes liver disease, including several disorders and diseases, such as cirrhosis or hepatitis that impair liver function.

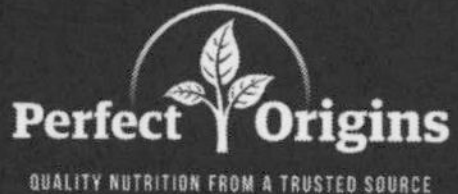

References:

Abenavoli, L., Capasso, R., Milic, N. and Capasso, F. (2010), Milk thistle in liver diseases: past, present, future. Phytother. Res., 24: 1423–1432. doi: 10.1002/ptr.3207

Awasthi, YC. Et al. (1998). Mechanisms of anticarcinogenic properties of curcumin: the effects of curcumin on glutathionelinked detoxification enzymes in rat liver.

Bustamante, J. et al. (1998). A-Lipoic Acid in Liver Metabolism and Disease. Free Radical Biology and Medicine. Volume 24, Issue 6. Pp. 1023-1039.

Cho, C.W. et al. (2010). Hypolipidemic and Antioxidant Effects of Dandelion Root and Leaf on Cholesterol-Fed Rabbits. International Journal of Molecular Science. 11, 67-78.

Kelly, G.S. (1998). Clinical Applications of N-Acetylcysteine. Alternative Medicine Review. Volume 3, No. 2.

Lin SC, et al. Hepatoprotective effects of Arctium lappa linne on liver injuries induced by chronic ethanol consumption and potentiated by carbon tetrachloride. J Biomed Sci 2002; 9:401

http://lpi.oregonstate.edu/infocenter/othernuts/choline/

http://www.liversupport.com/wordpress/2008/05/n-acetyl-cysteine-is-a-liver%E2%80%99s-ally/

Hepatoprotective activities of picroliv, curcumin, and ellagic acid compared to silymarin on carbon-tetrachloride-induced liver toxicity in mice

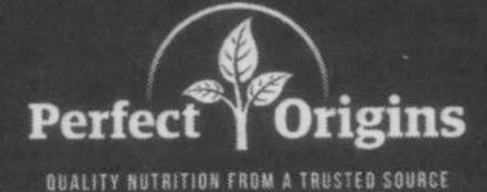

http://www.jpharmacol.com/article.asp?issn=0976-500X;year=2012;volume=3;issue=2;spage=149;epage=155;aulast=Girish

Daily Lemon Water

Start every day with warm lemon water. NOTE: This is NOT the Master Cleanse Lemonade Water. This is simply, a half of lemon squeezed in a cup of water. (Pinch of cayenne added if desired) Note that "warm" means room temperature and does not mean you need to warm the water on the stove or in the microwave. Also—and this is optional but highly encouraged—include a pinch of cayenne pepper powder. For an 8-ounce glass of water, use 1/2 lemon. End every day by drinking warm lemon water. Before bed warm lemon water with a pinch of cayenne pepper powder.

This will help stimulate your liver first thing in the morning, helping to cleanse it and promote detoxification. It also stimulates bowel movement, which is essential to aid in detoxification. It also helps stimulate bile production and the vitamin C content helps the liver synthesize toxins into a water-soluble substance for easy removal by the body.

Other benefits of warm lemon water are:

Aids in digestion and waste excretion

Promotes immune system and heart health

Rich in beneficial calcium and potassium minerals

Warm water is ideal to use because it helps with digestion. The liver can process and filter food much easier with warm water, thus reducing the amount of toxins, food particles, and contaminants that are released into the bloodstream.

The vitamin C in lemon juice works as an antioxidant, neutralizing the effect of free radicals in the body.

Alternative To Morning Lemon Water: Instead of drinking lemon water in the morning, use greens powder also. Greens powder is packed full of powdered vegetables and some fruits, vitamins, minerals, herbs, and probiotics. Using greens powder is a key ingredient in alkalizing your body.

Lemon Water Ingredients

Juice of ½ lemon or lime (preferably fresh squeezed and organic). Never use lemon juice from the bottle or frozen juice concentrate. (Save other half of lemon for next serving) Fresh squeezed lemons are full of enzymes that are good for your body!

1/10 teaspoon cayenne pepper (red pepper) natural or organic. Buy the flakes or powder in the spice

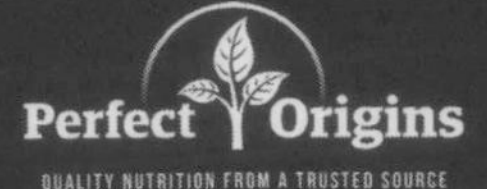

isle of the grocery store. If you can tolerate it, keep adding more. Red pepper has great thermogenic effects.

Eight ounces of water

Master Cleanse (Optional)

The Master Cleanse is an **OPTIONAL** cleanse that is cheap and practical. It was developed in the 1950's by a man named Stanley Burroughs. He has had great clinical success with it for all kinds of health issues. If you want to know more, you can google Master Cleanse and find a plethora of information on it. (Good and bad info. When researching alternative health topics, you will always find a bunch of negative information from supposed "experts". Remember that you can't judge everything by "double blind scientific research" those type of studies are extremely expensive and a lot of non-medical protocols don't have the money to run a trial like this.) The Master Cleanse lasts three to ten days and can provide the following benefits:

Dissolves and eliminates toxins and congestion

Reduces body fat by two to eight ounces per day

Cleanses the kidneys, liver and digestive system

Purifies the glands and cells

Eliminates waste and hardened material in the joints and muscles

Relieves pressure and irritation in the nerves, arteries, and blood vessels

Builds a healthy bloodstream

There are essentially 3 parts to the Master Cleanse.

1. Herbal Laxative Tea
2. Salt Water Flush
3. Lemonade

These will be discussed below:

Herbal Laxative Tea

To aid in the digestive system flush, purchase herbal laxative tea. Most health food stores and some grocery stores carry them. Drink one serving the evening before you start the cleanse. Here is one that works (but you can use another one) "Smooth Move" by Traditional Medicinals.

Saltwater Flush

The saltwater flush is a cheap, easy, controlled laxative that will cleanse your colon.

Prepare a full quart (four cups) of warm water, and add two level teaspoons of **uniodized sea salt** (iodized salt will not work properly).

Drink the entire quart preparation within 10 to 20 minutes. This will begin the process of thoroughly washing the entire digestive tract.

Do this as soon as you get up in the morning every day during the Master Cleanse.

The breaking up, loosening, and purging of encrusted debris from the small and large intestinal walls is the most important part of the Master Cleanse. You will need to use the bathroom throughout the flush. You should have two to three bowel movements per day.

For those readers who are concerned about blood pressure deviation due to salt ingestion, the uniodized salt and water have the same specific gravity as the blood; therefore, the kidneys cannot absorb the water, and the blood cannot absorb the salt. Hence, there is no salt retention. This saltwater flush may be performed as often as needed for proper washing of the entire digestive tract.

Perform this saltwater flush every day in the morning while you are on the cleanse, and remember that you will be saltwater flushing for the first hour of the day.

After the saltwater flush, begin taking the lemonade drink. During waking hours, drink eight, 8 ounce glasses of lemonade per day for a continuous purging of impurities from the digestive tract.

Lemonade

The lemonade is created by taking:

Juice of ½ lemon

2 Tablespoons of maple syrup

8 oz. of spring water

Pinch of cayenne pepper

Mix all of this together and drink within 10 minutes. There are live enzymes in this from the lemon that will die off within 10 minutes.

Steps to Perform the Master Cleanse

1. The night before you start the Master Cleanse, take a laxative tea such as *Smooth Move*, or get *Regular Tea* by Yogi Tea. It can be found at Kroger or Whole Foods.

2. Perform the saltwater flush early the next morning.

   Add two teaspoons of **uniodized sea salt** to four cups of lukewarm water. DO NOT USE IODIZED SALT!!!

   Drink all within 20 minutes.

   Perform this flush in the morning every day of the cleanse.

3. Drink lemonade eight times a day. (REMEMBER: This is NOT the same as daily lemon water that we talked about earlier - The master cleanse lemonade is designed for a cleanse)

   Squeeze ½ lemon into one cup of spring water.

   Add one to two tablespoons grade B pure maple syrup. (GRADE A can be used, but GRADE B maple syrup has more vitamins and minerals)

   Add a pinch of cayenne pepper powder.

   NOTE: if you want to drink more than 8 glasses a day of the lemonade, then go ahead! Drink more especially if you are active and choose to do exercise.

4. Repeat the Master Cleanse daily, including the salt water flush and the laxative tea at night for the

length of time you have decided to do the Master Cleanse - from 3 to 10 days. I personally recommend three days on the cleanse, and then three days off eating the Raw/Alkaline Diet, and then three days on the cleanse. Another option between the three day break is eating soups, and easy to digest foods. Avoid meat, wheat, dairy and sugar during this three day break!

If you must eat, the following foods contain lots of water and will be OK. Use restraint, however, because eating slows down the cleansing process.

Cucumbers
Watermelons
Oranges
Grapefruits
Celery
Tomatoes
Seedless grapes
Any type of fresh squeezed vegetable juice

You can also drink organic herbal teas throughout the day.

Master Cleanse Success Tips

Performing the Master Cleanse will be painful mentally because we are emotionally linked to food, and we have been trained all our lives to eat meat and carbohydrates at every meal. Eating non-organic, store-bought meat is very hard on your body and is linked to many health problems. You can get plenty of protein without meat.

If you cheat on the cleanse. That's OK, try again later. This program is designed to help you lose large amounts of weight in small steps.

There is no such thing as failure, just feedback. Don't be afraid to fail. Accept it, move on and persevere. Remember: BABY STEPS!

Stay strong and remember that you will eventually have your favorite foods again. You do have the will power to wait two to three weeks.

Use Perfect Flush to maximize your cleanse results. You can take this with any meal.

Cleansing Side Effects

During the cleanse, you may experience detoxification symptoms such as headaches, nausea, acne, low energy, bad odor, bad breath, or white tongue. This is actually good news. It means you are purging toxins from your body. You are getting better!

Use peppermint oil by:

Massaging several drops of peppermint essential oil on the abdomen, placing a drop on wrists, or inhaling to soothe the minor stomach discomfort associated with travel.

Rubbing one drop of peppermint essential oil on the temples, forehead, over the sinuses (careful to avoid contact with your eyes), and on the back of the neck to relieve head pressure.

You can drink mint tea to combat detoxification symptoms.

These will not slow down the detox process.

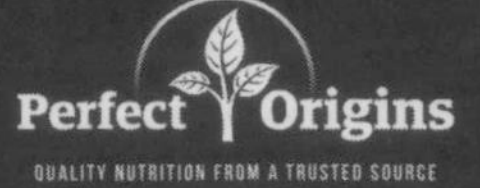

Raw / Alkaline Foods Diet

Why raw foods?

Raw fruits, vegetables, nuts and seeds are all chock full of nutrients. What specifically sets them apart is the fact that they have live enzymes in them that naturally heal and repair your body. When you cook food, you start to kill off the nutrition and the enzymes. This is where the term "enriched" comes in. Whenever you see that word on your food labels, it means that they've taken the nutrition out of the food and then had to put it back in, hence "enrich" it.

So what makes a food acid or alkaline? There are several things, but the most important rules are:

If a food is high in alkaline minerals including magnesium, potassium, calcium or sodium, it is likely to be alkaline to the body.

BUT – regardless of its alkaline mineral content, if any of the following are true, then it will be acidifying:

- Contains sugar
- Contains yeast
- Is fermented (like soy sauce)
- Contains fungi (like mushrooms)

Is refined, microwaved, or processed

The below chart is for those trying to "adjust" their body's pH level. The pH scale is from 0 to 14, with levels below 7 being acidic (low on oxygen) and numbers above 7 alkaline. An acidic body is a sickness and a "fat magnet." What you eat and drink will impact where your body's pH level falls. Balance is Key!

NOTE: For the next one to two weeks your goal should be 90-100% raw foods picked from the alkaline foods list below.

...ALKALINE FOODS...	...ACIDIC FOODS...
ALKALIZING VEGETABLES	ACIDIFYING VEGETABLES
Alfalfa	Corn
Barley Grass	Lentils
Beet Greens	Olives
Beets	Winter Squash
Broccoli	ACIDIFYING FRUITS
Cabbage	Blueberries

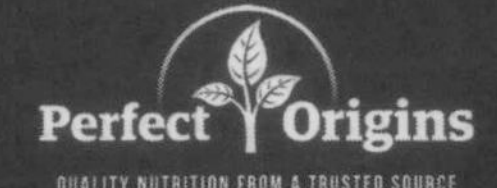

...ALKALINE FOODS...	...ACIDIC FOODS...
Carrot	Canned or Glazed Fruits
Cauliflower	Cranberries
Celery	Currants
Chard Greens	Plums**
Chlorella	Prunes**
Collard Greens	ACIDIFYING GRAINS, GRAIN PRODUCTS
Cucumber	Amaranth
Dandelions	Barley
Dulce	Bran, oat
Edible Flowers	Bran, wheat
Eggplant	Bread
Fermented Veggies	Corn
Garlic	Cornstarch
Green Beans	Crackers, soda
Green Peas	Flour, wheat
Kale	Flour, white
Kohlrabi	Hemp Seed Flour
Lettuce	Kamut
Mushrooms	Macaroni
Mustard Greens	Noodles
Nightshade Veggies	Oatmeal
Onions	Oats (rolled)
Parsnips (high glycemic)	Quinoa
Peas	Rice (all)
Peppers	Rice Cakes

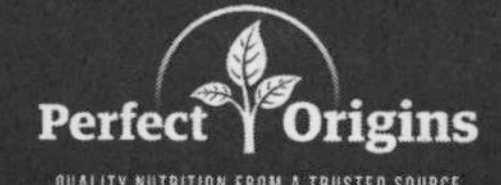

...ALKALINE FOODS...	...ACIDIC FOODS...
Pumpkin	Rye
Radishes	Spaghetti
Rutabaga	Spelt
Sea Veggies	Wheat Germ
Spinach, green	Wheat
Spirulina	ACIDIFYING BEANS & LEGUMES
Sprouts	Almond Milk
Sweet Potatoes	Black Beans
Tomatoes	Chick Peas
Watercress	Green Peas
Wheat Grass	Kidney Beans
Wild Greens	Lentils
ALKALIZING ORIENTAL VEGETABLES	Pinto Beans
Daikon	Red Beans
Dandelion Root	Rice Milk
Kombu	Soy Beans
Maitake	Soy Milk
Nori	White Beans
Reishi	ACIDIFYING DAIRY
Shitake	Butter
Umeboshi	Cheese
Wakame	Cheese, Processed
ALKALIZING FRUITS	Ice Cream
Apple	Ice Milk
Apricot	ACIDIFYING NUTS & BUTTERS

...ALKALINE FOODS...	...ACIDIC FOODS...
Avocado	Cashews
Banana (high glycemic)	Legumes
Berries	Peanut Butter
Blackberries	Peanuts
Cantaloupe	Pecans
Cherries, sour	Tahini
Coconut, fresh	Walnuts
Currants	ACIDIFYING ANIMAL PROTEIN
Dates, dried	Bacon
Figs, dried	Beef
Grapes	Carp
Grapefruit	Clams
Honeydew Melon	Cod
Lemon	Corned Beef
Lime	Fish
Muskmelons	Haddock
Nectarine	Lamb
Orange	Lobster
Peach	Mussels
Pear	Organ Meats
Pineapple	Oyster
Raisins	Pike
Raspberries	Pork
Rhubarb	Rabbit
Strawberries	Salmon

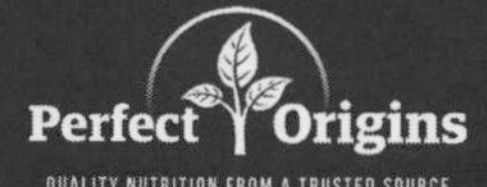

...ALKALINE FOODS...	...ACIDIC FOODS...
Tangerine	Sardines
Tomato	Sausage
Tropical Fruits	Scallops
Umeboshi Plums	Shellfish
Watermelon	Shrimp
ALKALIZING PROTEIN	Tuna
Almonds	Turkey
Chestnuts	Veal
Millet	Venison
Tempeh (fermented)	ACIDIFYING FATS & OILS
Tofu (fermented)	Avocado Oil
Whey Protein Powder	Butter
ALKALIZING SWEETENERS	Canola Oil
Stevia	Corn Oil
ALKALIZING SPICES & SEASONINGS	Flax Oil
Chili Pepper	Hemp Seed Oil
Cinnamon	Lard
Curry	Olive Oil
Ginger	Safflower Oil
Herbs (all)	Sesame Oil
Miso	Sunflower Oil
Mustard	ACIDIFYING SWEETENERS
Sea Salt	Carob
Tamari	Corn Syrup
ALKALIZING OTHER	Sugar

...ALKALINE FOODS...	...ACIDIC FOODS...
Alkaline Antioxidant Water	Nutra-sweet
Apple Cider Vinegar	Aspartame
Bee Pollen	Sucralose
Fresh Fruit Juice	Neotame
Green Juices	ACIDIFYING ALCOHOL
Lecithin Granules	Beer
Mineral Water	Hard Liquor
Molasses, blackstrap	Spirits
Probiotic Cultures	Wine
Soured Dairy Products	ACIDIFYING OTHER FOODS
Veggie Juices	Catsup
ALKALIZING MINERALS	Cocoa
Calcium: pH 12	Coffee
Cesium: pH 14	Mustard
Magnesium: pH 9	Pepper
Potassium: pH 14	Soft Drinks
Sodium: pH 14	Vinegar

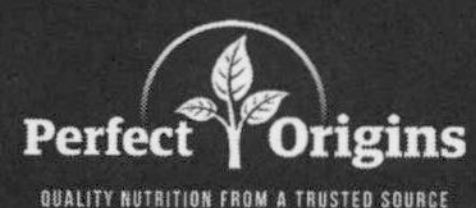

...ALKALINE FOODS...	...ACIDIC FOODS...
Although it might seem that citrus fruits would have an acidifying effect on the body, the citric acid they contain actually has an alkalinizing effect in the system. Note that a food's acid or alkaline forming tendency in the body has nothing to do with the actual pH of the food itself. For example, lemons are very acidic, however the end products they produce after digestion and assimilation are very alkaline so, lemons are alkaline forming in the body. Likewise, meat will test alkaline before digestion, but it leaves a very acidic residue in the body so, like nearly all animal products, meat is very acid forming.	ACIDIFYING DRUGS & CHEMICALS
	Aspirin
	Chemicals
	Drugs, Medicinal
	Drugs, Psychedelic
	Herbicides
	Pesticides
	Tobacco
	ACIDIFYING JUNK FOOD
	Beer: pH 2.5
	Coca-Cola: pH 2
	Coffee: pH 4
	** These foods leave an alkaline ash but have an acidifying effect on the body.

UNKNOWN:
There are several versions of the Acidic and Alkaline Food chart to be found in different books and on the Internet. The following foods are sometimes attributed to the acidic side of the chart and sometimes to the alkaline side. Remember, you don't need to adhere strictly to the alkaline side of the chart, just make sure a good percentage of the foods you eat come from the alkaline side. The foods below can be eaten in moderation.

Brazil Nuts	Maple Syrup
Brussel Sprouts	Milk
Buckwheat	Nuts
Cashews	Organic Milk (unpasteurized)
Chicken	Potatoes, white
Corn	Pumpkin Seeds
Cottage Cheese	Quinoa
Eggs	Sauerkraut

...ALKALINE FOODS...	...ACIDIC FOODS...
Flax Seeds	Soy Products
Green Tea	Sprouted Seeds
Herbal Tea	Squashes
Honey	Sunflower Seeds
Kombucha	Tomatoes
Lima Beans	Yogurt
* These statements have not been evaluated by the Food and Drug Administration and are not intended to diagnose, treat, cure, or prevent any disease; research is ongoing.	

Managing Fruits

Cut back on fruits!

Yes, I said it. You've heard all your life that fruits are healthy and help you lose weight. This is just a half truth. Here's the real story...

Fruit is full of fructose, which is much more readily transformed to fat inside the liver than glucose. So when you are eating a lot of fruit, it is being stored as fat. This could be the #1 reason why people who eat healthy can't lose weight. They are eating too much fruit! Fruit exits the liver as fat, so it doesn't cause those insulin spikes. It is also low glycemic, and contains fiber and lots of vitamins and minerals. I don't eliminate fruit from my diet, but I now eat It In moderatlon. Less than 100 grams a day.

The best way to approach this is to just eat more raw veggies and a little bit of fruit every day. One piece of fruit a day is best and unlimited raw vegetables. Your liver will be happier and your weight loss efforts more successful!

Structured Eating

Structured eating is a well-established approach to dieting and fat loss. The principles of structured eating are founded on the concept of *intermittent fasting*. If you are worried by the word "fasting"—possibly because you have never tried it before—don't be. Fasting is an excellent thing to do for your liver, your health and well-being in general. It has been practiced in biblical times, and even before then (mainly because they didn't have food).

As you may already know, hormones play a significant role in the process of weight management. Some hormones trigger fat-*burning* while others stimulate fat-*gaining*. When you fast, those hormones that promote fat-burning are stimulated and those that promote fat-gaining are suppressed. *Perfect Origins* presents specific diet plans that utilize the powerful tool of fasting.

The Structured Eating process can be divided into three components:

Structured Eating Level 1 – At this level, you maintain the same food intake and meals; however, you modify the intake times such that you consume the meals only between noon and 9pm.

Structured Eating Level 2 – At this level, you begin to add in foods in the list provided on pages 22-27, the alkaline list, or the grocery list I've given you below. Consume those healthy foods about 50% of the time.

Structured Eating Level 3 – At this level, you begin

to add in foods in the list provided on pages 22-27, alkaline list or the grocery list below. Consume about 90% of the time.

The more fat-burning foods you consume, the quicker you will see results. Although Structured Eating comes in various forms, this version leverages making the intelligent choices at the specific times. If you go out to eat for a hamburger, instead of adding tater tots, choose a salad. The plan you are on allows you to pick the tater tots, but making optimal and healthy choices at these decision points will bring faster results.

How Structured Eating Helps You Lose Weight

1. *A Burst of Energy Burns More Calories* – You will likely find that you are highly productive during your fasting period. This is because fasting for less than three days (72 hours) will increase your adrenaline level and ramp up your metabolism, in turn increasing the number of calories you burn. This extra energy may give you the boost you need for a workout or to get more of your daily tasks accomplished. All of this in turn leads to increased calorie burning.

2. *Burning Off Fats Rather Than Sugars* - The fasting process gives your body no choice but to burn stored fat. Any excess fat your body doesn't burn during the several hours after a meal is stored in fat cells. When you consume food, the body prefers to burn carbs and then

fat from the food, in that order. Fasting transforms the body's metabolism so it burns mostly fat instead of blood sugar. By the end of a 24-hour fast, your body is burning far more fat than it would during a regular day of eating.

3. *Consume the Foods You Like* - Short term fasting allows you to lose weight and burn fat without missing any of the foods you like. With short-term fasting, you can consume all the foods you like—when you want them—and without any guilt, and the fat still comes off.

4. *Increase the Hormones That Burn Fat* – Hormones control your body's core metabolic functions, with growth hormone being the most critical fat-burning hormone in the body.. When you fast, insulin levels decrease, thus you burn body fat rather than store it. Growth hormone production also accelerates and the fat burning operations step into high hear.

5. *Increase Fat Burning Enzyme Levels* - Fasting increases the activity of two key fat burning enzymes. *Hormone Sensitive Lipase* triggers the fat cells to release fat, which in turn becomes energy to the muscles. *Lipoprotein Lipase* induces the muscle cells to take up fat, which in turn is burned as fuel. Fasting boosts both of these enzymes, and the end result is fat burning.

6. *You Discover What Causes You to Eat* – Fasting gives you an entirely new perspective on what causes you to eat. When you stop eating for a day, your various reasons for eating are laid bare. This psychological revelation becomes the most effective step to removing all your bad eating habits.

7. *Builds a Positive Attitude* - Each fast, however small, becomes an accomplishment that builds confidence. You feel good about your accomplishments and you come to like your relationship with food again. Each successful fast

builds on the last, and ultimately you regain control over your food choices.

8. *Detoxes Your Liver* – On a daily basis, your poor little liver is bombard by toxins. Toxic substances that are in the foods you eat, air you breathe, lotions you put on your skin, even the water that you drink.

Your liver is constantly working overtime to destroy these unwanted toxins and protect the body from harm. Even healthy individuals should be fasting to keep their liver working at its best. Why not give it a break? This small rest period allows your liver to "de stress". In the toxic world that we live in, it is inevitable that we deal with processing heavy amounts of toxins daily. Fasting is an easy way to boost your health and metabolism, not to mention your energy levels ☺!

Eating for fat loss doesn't need to be complicated and food should never be a source of anxiety or guilt. Mixing a few 24-hour fasts or daily 15 hour fasts (9pm-12pm) into your week can liberate you from the dieting drudge and allow you to enjoy food again.

Serving Sizes:

6-8 oz of proteins

1 cup of carbs (beans, rice, etc)

1 cup of veggies

½ cup of fruits

¼ cup of healthy fats

everything else… small amounts

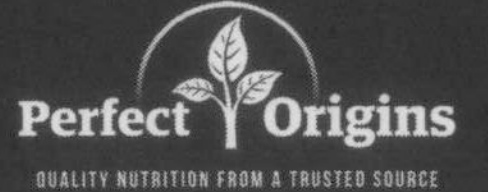

STRUCTURED EATING GROCERY LIST

Eat foods in red 1 serving every other day. HONEY should only be eaten every 3 to 4 days if at all. Avoid it as much as possible

CARBOHYDRATES

COMPLEX/STARCHY

- ☐ oats
- ☐ wild rice
- ☐ jasmine rice (white rice)
- ☐ basmati rice
- ☐ quinoa

STARCHY VEGGIES

- ☐ yams
- ☐ sweet potatoes
- ☐ red/white potatoes (limited)
- ☐ beans,lentils,legumes (limited)
- ☐ carrots
- ☐ squash

FIBROUS VEGGIES

- ☐ alfalfa
- ☐ artichoke
- ☐ arugula
- ☐ bean sprouts
- ☐ bamboo shoots
- ☐ broccoli
- ☐ beets
- ☐ brussel sprouts
- ☐ cabbage (red, green)
- ☐ celery
- ☐ cauliflower

PROTEINS

RED MEAT

- ☐ grass fed beef
- ☐ venison/deer
- ☐ lean ground beef
- ☐ lamb
- ☐ bison
- ☐ elk (any wild game)

POULTRY

free range is best

- ☐ chicken breast
- ☐ ground chicken
- ☐ turkey breast
- ☐ ground turkey

FISH

- ☐ wild salmon (not atlantic)
- ☐ tuna
- ☐ mahimahi
- ☐ swordfish
- ☐ whitefish
- ☐ sea bass
- ☐ grouper
- ☐ snapper
- ☐ trout
- ☐ mackerel
- ☐ halibut

- ☐ broccoli
- ☐ beets
- ☐ brussel sprouts
- ☐ cabbage (red, green)
- ☐ celery
- ☐ cauliflower
- ☐ cucumber
- ☐ green beans
- ☐ kale/mustard greens
- ☐ lettuce (all kinds)
- ☐ onions
- ☐ parsley/cilantro
- ☐ pepper (all kinds)
- ☐ okra
- ☐ mushrooms
- ☐ radishes
- ☐ seaweed
- ☐ swiss chard
- ☐ snow peas/snap peas
- ☐ spinach
- ☐ string beans
- ☐ tomato
- ☐ turnips
- ☐ watercress
- ☐ wheatgrass
- ☐ zuchini
- ☐ bok choy
- ☐ squash (summer/winter)
- ☐ collard greens
- ☐ asparagus
- ☐ sea vegetables

NATURAL SIMPLE

- ☐ apples (all kinds)
- ☐ berries (all kinds)
- ☐ strawberries
- ☐ blueberries
- ☐ blackberries
- ☐ raspberries
- ☐ grapes
- ☐ grapefruit
- ☐ kiwi
- ☐ lemons
- ☐ limes
- ☐ pineapple
- ☐ pears
- ☐ mangoes
- ☐ nectarines

- ☐ sea bass
- ☐ grouper
- ☐ snapper
- ☐ trout
- ☐ mackerel
- ☐ halibut
- ☐ rainbow trout
- ☐ cod
- ☐ sardines
- ☐ scallops
- ☐ shrimp
- ☐ tilapia

EGGS

- ☐ cage free

BEANS (limited)

(protein & carb)

- ☐ white
- ☐ lima
- ☐ chickpeas
- ☐ navy
- ☐ pinto
- ☐ kidney
- ☐ red beans
- ☐ black beans
- ☐ hummus
- ☐ lentils

NUTS (raw)

(protein & fat)

- ☐ almonds
- ☐ walnuts
- ☐ pine nuts
- ☐ hazel nuts
- ☐ cashews
- ☐ macadamia

SEEDS raw

(protein & fat)

- ☐ pumpkin
- ☐ sunflower
- ☐ chia
- ☐ flax
- ☐ hemp

- ☐ oranges
- ☐ dates
- ☐ plums
- ☐ watermelon
- ☐ cantaloupe
- ☐ figs

CONDIMENTS

- ☐ almond butter
- ☐ tahini
- ☐ herbs
- ☐ kerry gold unsalted butter
- ☐ apple cider vinegar
- ☐ Bragg's liquid aminos
- ☐ ginger
- ☐ balsalmic vinegrette
- ☐ all natural salsa
- ☐ all natural hot sauce (Frank's)
- ☐ spices without msg
- ☐ olive oil based
- ☐ chemical free dressings
- ☐ natural peanut butter
- ☐ herbs
- ☐ ketchup(w/out hfcs)
- ☐ Mrs. Dash without salt

SWEETENERS

- ☐ sugar leaf
- ☐ HONEY
- ☐ Stevia/Stevia Plus
- ☐ maple syrup
- ☐ Eryrithritol, Xylitol

BEVERAGES

- ☐ water (spring, filtered)
- ☐ veggie juices
- ☐ coconut milk (unsweetened)
- ☐ herbal tea
- ☐ almond milk (unsweetened)
- ☐ hemp milk

FATS

- ☐ extra virgin olive oil
- ☐ coconut oil
- ☐ omega 3 fish oil
- ☐ cod liver oil
- ☐ chia seeds
- ☐ hemp seed
- ☐ krill oil
- ☐ avocados
- ☐ natural coconut flakes

SUPPLEMENTS

- ☐ BioTrust Protein Powder
- ☐ organic fiber
- ☐ greens powder
- ☐ multi vitamin
- ☐ Perfect Biotics Probiotic
- ☐ digestive enzyme
- ☐ Perfect Omega TG
- ☐ LivLean Formula #1

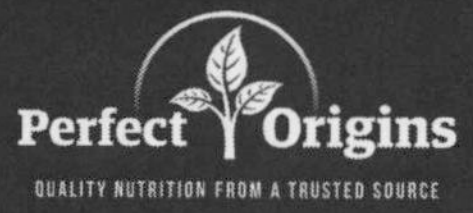

Cheat Day

On the day prior to the fasting, you can eat almost any food(s) you desire. We call this day the "Cheat Day" and the free eating continues until 8pm.

When the clock strikes 8pm, you will go into fasting mode and remain in this mode continuously for 24 hours. Remember this is the evening of your cheat day. The fasting continues while you are asleep and on into the next day, during which you can drink only steeped herbal teas or water.

The goal of the Cheat Day is to elevate the hormone leptin, which will signal the body to start burning fat. This is accomplished by calorie bombardment.

NOTE: If you want to move this time from 9pm to 10 or 11pm, go ahead! Just make sure that you get 24hrs in!

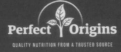

48-Hour Fast (Optional- For those that are hard core ;-))

The 48-Hour Fast is performed one time every other month and is optional for those who want extreme fat burning. During this time, you can have water, herbal teas, and chew gum. These three things are enough to get you through the fast.

The fast works extremely well. The below photographs illustrate my own personal results in 48 hrs. Notice how it took the swelling out of my belly.

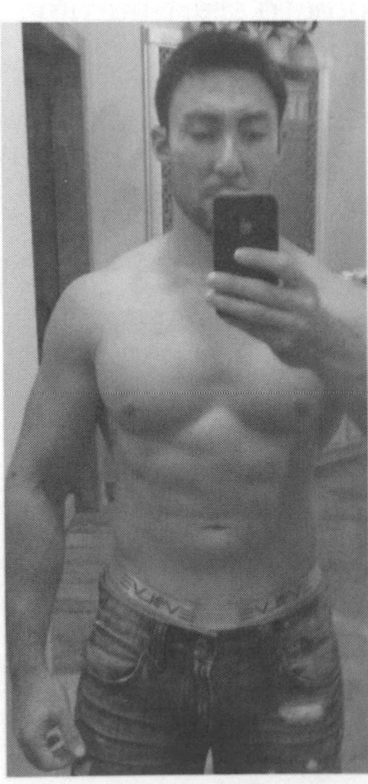

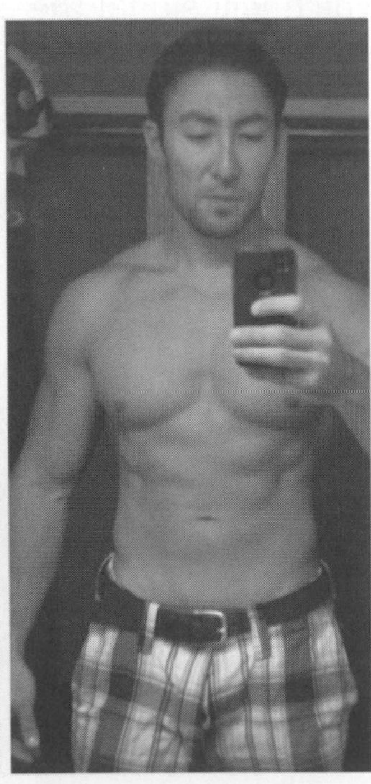

Well, I hope that you enjoyed the book. I want to leave you with this notion before we go:

Mindset Shift... Please Read!

To stay healthy, to lose weight, to gain muscle, to run farther, to run faster, to learn an instrument, to train for any type of event, all require one thing: Growth.

If you took 12 weeks and learned to play piano, by practicing every day for 30 minutes. In 12 weeks, you could play a few pieces of music.

What if you stopped? Eventually you would forget how to play. What if you trained for 3 months to run a mini marathon? Running every single day, building up to 13.1 miles.

You run the race, achieve your goal and then stop running. Do you think in 5 weeks, you could still run 13.1 miles even though you stopped running? No way!

The same goes for weight loss. If you spend 12 weeks to lose 30lbs and reach your goal. Then, you go right back to what you were eating before you started the diet and LivLean. Do you think you'd gain weight? ABSOLUTELY.

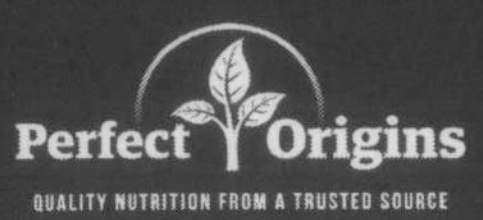

"Do what you've always done, and you'll get what you've always gotten."

The body is an amazingly adaptive organism and whatever you put into it, is exactly what you'll get out of it. Put garbage in, you will get garbage out!

If you have any questions what so ever, you can email my team and I at support@perfectorigins.com.

Good Luck and God Bless!

Dr Charles and Your Perfect Origins Wellness Team